MW01206530

Guide for Beginners

Understanding the Importance of Neurogenesis Diet

By

Mackenzie Naois

Table of Contents

CHAPTER 1 5

Introduction 5

1.1 What is Neurogenesis? 5

1.2 The Importance of Neurogenesis
....7

1.3 Why a Neurogenesis Diet? 9

CHAPTER 2 13

Understanding Neurogenesis...........13

2.1 The Science Behind
Neurogenesis 13

2.2 Neuroplasticity and Brain
Health 15

2.3 Factors Affecting Neurogenesis
....17

CHAPTER 3 21

Getting Started with the Neurogenesis
Diet 21

3.1 Assessing Your Current Diet..21

3.2 Setting Your Goals 23

3.3 Creating a Balanced Approach
....25

CHAPTER 4 29

Neurogenesis Diet Principles 29

4.1 Foods that Promote
Neurogenesis 29

4.2 Foods to Avoid or Limit.........34

4.3 Meal Planning and Timing.....39

CHAPTER 5 44

Neurogenesis Diet Recipes..............44

5.1 Breakfast Options...................44

5.2 Lunch Ideas 50

5.3 Dinner Recipes 57

5.4 Snacks and Smoothies............62

CHAPTER 6 66

Incorporating Lifestyle Changes 66

6.1 Exercise and Neurogenesis.....66

6.2 Sleep and Stress Management 72

6.3 Cognitive Stimulation 78

CHAPTER 7....................................85

Monitoring Your Progress...............85

7.1 Tracking Your Diet 85

7.2 Assessing Cognitive Changes 87

7.3 Adjusting Your Plan...............89

CHAPTER 1

Introduction

1.1 What is Neurogenesis?

Neurogenesis, a captivating and relatively recent discovery in neuroscience, refers to the process by which new neurons or nerve cells are generated from neural stem cells or progenitor cells in the brain. This process primarily occurs in two specific regions of the brain: the subgranular zone (SGZ) of the hippocampus and the subventricular zone (SVZ) lining the lateral ventricles. These newly formed neurons integrate into existing neural circuits, which can have profound implications for cognitive function, learning, memory, mood regulation, and overall brain health.

The concept of neurogenesis was once believed to be limited to early development and adolescence, with the notion that the adult brain's neuronal population remained relatively static throughout life. However, groundbreaking research in the late 20th and early 21st centuries has shattered this dogma. It has become abundantly clear that neurogenesis persists throughout adulthood and plays a pivotal role in maintaining brain plasticity and adaptability.

1.2 The Importance of Neurogenesis

The significance of neurogenesis cannot be overstated. It underscores the brain's remarkable ability to adapt and regenerate, offering hope for individuals of all ages. Here are some key reasons why neurogenesis is of paramount importance:

1. **Learning and Memory:** Neurogenesis is closely linked to cognitive functions such as learning and memory. New neurons in the hippocampus contribute to the formation of memories and the capacity to acquire new knowledge.

2. **Emotional Well-being:** Neurogenesis has a strong impact on emotional health and mood regulation. It is

associated with reduced symptoms of depression, anxiety, and stress. Antidepressant medications often enhance neurogenesis, highlighting the connection between mood disorders and neural regeneration.

3. **Brain Repair and Recovery:** In cases of brain injury or neurodegenerative diseases, neurogenesis offers a potential avenue for repair and recovery. While it may not fully reverse conditions like Alzheimer's disease, it can help mitigate some cognitive decline.

4. **Adaptation and Resilience:** Neurogenesis is a core component of brain plasticity, allowing the brain to adapt to new environments, experiences,

and challenges. This adaptability is crucial for long-term mental health and cognitive vitality.

1.3 Why a Neurogenesis Diet?

Now, you might wonder why a specific diet is necessary to support neurogenesis. The answer lies in the profound impact that nutrition has on brain health and, consequently, neurogenesis. A "Neurogenesis Diet" is designed to optimize the conditions within your body and brain to promote the generation of new neurons. Here's why it's essential:

1. **Nutrient Supply:** The brain demands a constant supply of essential nutrients to function

optimally. A neurogenesis diet focuses on providing the right balance of vitamins, minerals, antioxidants, and other nutrients that support the growth and survival of new neurons.

2. **Neuroprotective Effects:** Certain foods are rich in compounds like antioxidants and anti-inflammatory agents that protect existing neurons from damage and promote an environment conducive to neurogenesis.

3. **Hormonal Regulation:** Diet can influence hormones and growth factors like brain-derived neurotrophic factor (BDNF) and insulin-like growth factor 1 (IGF-1), which are critical for neurogenesis. A

neurogenesis diet can help regulate these factors.

4. **Gut-Brain Connection:** Emerging research indicates a strong connection between the gut microbiome and brain health. A neurogenesis diet can support a healthy gut, which in turn can positively affect neurogenesis and overall brain function.

a neurogenesis diet is a strategic approach to nourishing your brain, enhancing cognitive function, and promoting mental well-being by providing the nutrients and conditions that foster the birth of new neurons and the overall health of your brain. This introduction sets the stage for exploring the fascinating world of neurogenesis and how dietary choices can significantly impact our brain's capacity to thrive and adapt throughout our lives.

CHAPTER 2

Understanding Neurogenesis

2.1 The Science Behind Neurogenesis

Neurogenesis, the process of generating new neurons in the brain, is a remarkable and intricate biological phenomenon. Understanding the science behind neurogenesis is essential to appreciate its significance fully.

At its core, neurogenesis involves the transformation of neural stem cells or progenitor cells into mature, functional neurons. This process primarily occurs in two specialized regions of the brain: the subgranular zone (SGZ) of the hippocampus, a structure crucial for memory and learning, and the subventricular zone (SVZ), lining the lateral ventricles. Here's a simplified overview of the steps involved:

1. **Proliferation:** Neural stem cells divide and produce progenitor cells.

2. **Differentiation:** Progenitor cells differentiate into immature neurons.

3. **Migration:** Immature neurons move to their designated locations within the brain.

4. **Integration:** Immature neurons mature into functional neurons and integrate into existing neural circuits.

Several key factors influence this process, including genetic and environmental factors, age, and overall brain health.

2.2 Neuroplasticity and Brain Health

Neurogenesis is closely intertwined with the concept of neuroplasticity, which refers to the brain's ability to adapt and reorganize itself in response to experiences, learning, and environmental changes. Neuroplasticity encompasses not only the formation of new neurons but also the rewiring of existing neural pathways.

Neuroplasticity is essential for brain health and cognitive function throughout life. It enables us to acquire new skills, recover from brain injuries, and adapt to changing circumstances. Neurogenesis plays a vital role in this process by providing a constant supply of fresh neurons that can be incorporated into existing networks, enhancing cognitive flexibility and adaptability.

The relationship between neuroplasticity and neurogenesis highlights the brain's remarkable capacity to learn, adapt, and recover. It also underscores the potential for interventions that support neurogenesis to improve brain health, combat cognitive decline, and enhance overall well-being.

2.3 Factors Affecting Neurogenesis

Neurogenesis is a dynamic process influenced by a range of factors, both intrinsic and extrinsic. Here are some key elements that can impact neurogenesis:

1. **Age:** Neurogenesis is most robust during early development and declines with age. However, it continues to occur throughout adulthood, albeit at a reduced rate. Strategies that support neurogenesis become increasingly important as we age.

2. **Physical Activity:** Regular exercise has been shown to boost neurogenesis by increasing the production of

growth factors like brain-derived neurotrophic factor (BDNF). Aerobic exercise, in particular, has a positive impact on brain health.

3. **Diet and Nutrition:** Certain dietary components, such as antioxidants, omega-3 fatty acids, and flavonoids, can support neurogenesis by providing the necessary building blocks and protecting neurons from damage.

4. **Stress and Cortisol:** Chronic stress and elevated cortisol levels can inhibit neurogenesis. Stress management techniques, such as mindfulness and relaxation exercises, may help mitigate this effect.

5. **Sleep:** Quality sleep is crucial for neurogenesis and overall brain health. During sleep, the brain consolidates memories and undergoes repair processes that support the growth of new neurons.

6. **Environmental Enrichment:** An intellectually stimulating environment with exposure to novel experiences can enhance neurogenesis by promoting the formation of new neural connections.

7. **Neurological Disorders:** Certain neurological conditions, such as depression and Alzheimer's disease, are associated with reduced neurogenesis. Therapies that promote neurogenesis are a

focus of research in these fields.

These factors and their impact on neurogenesis is essential for individuals seeking to optimize their brain health and cognitive function. By making informed lifestyle choices and incorporating strategies that support neurogenesis, we can harness the brain's innate capacity for growth and adaptation throughout our lives.

CHAPTER 3

Getting Started with the Neurogenesis Diet

3.1 Assessing Your Current Diet

Embarking on the journey of a Neurogenesis Diet begins with a critical self-assessment of your current dietary habits. This step is essential because it helps you identify areas that need improvement and provides a baseline for tracking your progress. Here's how to assess your current diet:

- **Food Journal:** Keep a detailed record of everything you eat and drink for a few days or a week. Include portion sizes and note the timing of your meals.

- **Nutrient Analysis:** Analyze your food journal to assess the nutritional content of your diet. Pay attention to key nutrients such as vitamins, minerals, fiber, healthy fats, and protein.

- **Identify Problem Areas:** Look for patterns in your eating habits. Are you consuming too much processed food, sugar, or unhealthy fats? Are you getting enough fruits and vegetables? Are you staying hydrated?

- **Consider Special Diets:** If you have specific dietary restrictions or follow a particular diet (e.g., vegetarian, vegan, gluten-free), evaluate how these choices align with the principles of the Neurogenesis Diet.

3.2 Setting Your Goals

Once you've assessed your current diet, it's time to set clear and achievable goals for your Neurogenesis Diet journey. Goals provide direction and motivation for making positive dietary changes. Here's how to set effective goals:

- **Specific and Measurable:** Define your goals in a specific and measurable way. For example, instead of saying, "I want to eat healthier," specify, "I will eat at least three servings of vegetables every day."

- **Realistic and Attainable:** Ensure your goals are realistic and attainable based on your current lifestyle and dietary habits. Gradual changes are often more sustainable than drastic ones.

- **Time-Bound:** Set a timeframe for achieving your goals. This could be weekly, monthly, or quarterly. Having a timeline helps you stay accountable.

- **Prioritize:** Identify which aspects of your diet need the most attention and prioritize those goals. For example, if you consume excessive sugar, your primary goal might be to reduce added sugar intake.

- **Write Them Down:** Putting your goals in writing increases your commitment to them. Create a list of your dietary goals and review them regularly.

3.3 Creating a Balanced Approach

A balanced approach to the Neurogenesis Diet is crucial to ensure that you receive a wide range of nutrients and maintain a sustainable eating plan. Here are some principles to guide you:

- **Variety:** Incorporate a diverse range of foods from all food groups. This ensures that you receive a wide array of nutrients and phytochemicals that support brain health.

- **Moderation:** Avoid extremes and practice portion control. Overindulging in even healthy foods can lead to unwanted consequences.

- **Whole Foods:** Emphasize whole, minimally processed foods over highly processed and refined options. Whole grains, fresh fruits and vegetables, lean proteins, and healthy fats should form the basis of your diet.

- **Hydration:** Stay adequately hydrated by drinking plenty of water throughout the day. Dehydration can negatively affect cognitive function.

- **Mindful Eating:** Pay attention to your body's hunger and fullness cues. Mindful eating promotes a healthier relationship with food and can prevent overeating.

- **Meal Planning:** Plan your meals and snacks in advance to make it easier to stick to your dietary goals. Prepare healthy options to have readily available.

- **Seek Professional Guidance:** If you have specific dietary concerns or medical conditions, consider consulting a registered dietitian or healthcare professional for personalized guidance.

Assessing your current diet, setting achievable goals, and adopting a balanced approach, you can lay a strong foundation for your Neurogenesis Diet journey.

Remember that making lasting dietary changes is a gradual process, and consistency is key to reaping the long-term benefits of improved brain health and overall well-being.

CHAPTER 4

Neurogenesis Diet Principles

4.1 Foods that Promote Neurogenesis

The Neurogenesis Diet is centered around the consumption of foods that support the growth and development of new neurons while providing overall brain health benefits. Incorporating these neurogenesis-promoting foods into your daily meals can be a proactive step towards enhancing cognitive function and maintaining brain health. Here's a list of foods that are known to promote neurogenesis:

1. Fatty Fish: Fatty fish like salmon, trout, mackerel, and sardines are rich in omega-3 fatty acids, particularly docosahexaenoic acid (DHA). DHA is a key component of brain cell membranes and is associated with improved cognitive function and neurogenesis.

2. Blueberries: Blueberries are packed with antioxidants, specifically flavonoids like anthocyanins, which have been linked to enhanced learning capacity and neurogenesis. They also help reduce oxidative stress in the brain.

3. Dark Leafy Greens: Vegetables like spinach, kale, and Swiss chard are abundant sources of folate, a B-vitamin that plays a role in DNA synthesis and repair, supporting the growth of new neurons.

4. Turmeric: Curcumin, the active compound in turmeric, has potent anti-inflammatory and antioxidant properties. It may contribute to neurogenesis and protect against neurodegenerative diseases.

5. Broccoli: Broccoli and other cruciferous vegetables contain sulforaphane, a compound known for its neuroprotective effects. It may enhance cognitive function and support brain health.

6. Nuts and Seeds: Walnuts, almonds, flaxseeds, and chia seeds are rich in healthy fats, antioxidants, and vitamins, providing essential nutrients for brain health and neurogenesis.

7. Berries: Besides blueberries, strawberries, raspberries, and blackberries contain various antioxidants and phytochemicals that can support brain health and potentially boost neurogenesis.

8. Dark Chocolate: High-quality dark chocolate with a cocoa content of 70% or higher contains flavonoids that may improve cognitive function, increase blood flow to the brain, and support neurogenesis in moderation.

9. Green Tea: Epigallocatechin gallate (EGCG) in green tea is a powerful antioxidant that may enhance cognitive function and neurogenesis. It also provides a modest caffeine boost for alertness.

10. Whole Grains: Whole grains like oats, quinoa, and brown rice provide a steady supply of complex carbohydrates, fiber, and essential nutrients, which help maintain stable blood sugar levels and support brain function.

11. Avocado: Avocado is rich in healthy monounsaturated fats, which support overall brain health and may contribute to neurogenesis. It also contains vitamins and minerals important for brain function.

12. Eggs: Eggs are a source of choline, a nutrient that plays a role in the production of acetylcholine, a neurotransmitter involved in memory and learning. Choline supports brain health and potentially neurogenesis.

13. Berries: Besides blueberries, strawberries, raspberries, and blackberries contain various antioxidants and phytochemicals that can support brain health and potentially boost neurogenesis.

14. Beans and Legumes: These foods are excellent sources of complex carbohydrates, fiber, and plant-based protein. They provide a steady release of energy and support brain function.

4.2 Foods to Avoid or Limit

While incorporating neurogenesis-promoting foods into your diet is essential, it's equally important to be mindful of foods that can hinder or negatively impact the process of neurogenesis. Here is a list of foods that you should avoid or limit when following a Neurogenesis Diet:

1. Sugar and High-Fructose Corn Syrup: Excessive sugar intake, especially from sources like sugary beverages, candies, and processed foods, can lead to inflammation, insulin resistance, and impaired neurogenesis. High-fructose corn syrup is particularly detrimental to brain health.

2. Trans Fats: Artificial trans fats found in partially hydrogenated oils are linked to cognitive decline and inflammation. Avoid fried foods and processed snacks containing trans fats.

3. Highly Processed Foods: Processed foods often contain additives, preservatives, and artificial flavorings that may have adverse effects on brain health. Opt for whole, minimally processed foods whenever possible.

4. Excessive Saturated Fat: While some saturated fat is necessary for brain health, excessive consumption from sources like red meat and full-fat dairy products can increase the risk of cognitive decline. Limit your intake of these foods.

5. Alcohol: Excessive alcohol consumption can harm brain cells, impair cognitive function, and inhibit neurogenesis. If you choose to consume alcohol, do so in moderation.

6. Refined Grains: Foods made from refined grains, such as white bread, white rice, and sugary cereals, can lead to rapid spikes in blood sugar levels, which may negatively affect neurogenesis. Opt for whole grains instead.

7. Artificial Sweeteners: Some studies suggest that artificial sweeteners like aspartame may disrupt gut microbiota and have adverse effects on brain health. Use them sparingly, if at all.

8. High-Sodium Foods: Excessive salt intake can lead to high blood pressure, which is associated with cognitive decline. Limit your consumption of highly salted foods and processed snacks.

9. Processed Meats: Processed meats like bacon, sausages, and deli meats often contain unhealthy additives and preservatives. High consumption is linked to an increased risk of neurodegenerative diseases.

10. Excessive Caffeine: While moderate caffeine consumption can have cognitive benefits, excessive caffeine intake can disrupt sleep patterns and lead to increased stress, potentially hindering neurogenesis. Be mindful of your caffeine intake, especially later in the day.

11. Artificial Additives: Some artificial food additives, such as monosodium glutamate (MSG) and artificial food colorings, have been associated with adverse effects on brain health in sensitive individuals. Read food labels to identify and avoid these additives.

12. Excessively Salty Foods: A high-sodium diet can lead to elevated blood pressure, which is associated with cognitive decline. Reduce your intake of excessively salty foods, such as fast food and heavily processed snacks.

13. Chronic Overeating: Excessive calorie intake beyond your body's energy needs can lead to obesity, insulin resistance, and inflammation, all of which can negatively impact neurogenesis. Practice portion control and mindful eating.

moderation is key when it comes to foods to limit or avoid. A Neurogenesis Diet focuses on providing the brain with the best possible nutrients and environment for neurogenesis, which means making informed choices about both what to include and what to limit in your diet.

4.3 Meal Planning and Timing

Meal planning and timing play a significant role in the effectiveness of a Neurogenesis Diet. By structuring your meals and considering the timing of your food intake, you can optimize nutrient absorption, stabilize blood sugar levels, and support neurogenesis. Here are some guidelines for meal planning and timing on a Neurogenesis Diet:

1. Regular Meals: Aim to eat regular meals throughout the day, including breakfast, lunch, and dinner. Skipping meals or going too long without eating can lead to fluctuations in blood sugar levels, which can negatively affect cognitive function.

2. Balanced Macronutrients: Each meal should ideally include a balance of macronutrients—carbohydrates, proteins, and fats. This balance helps provide a steady release of energy and supports brain health.

3. Include Neurogenesis-Promoting Foods: Incorporate foods that promote neurogenesis, as mentioned in section 4.1, into your meals and snacks. Try to include a variety of these foods in your diet.

4. Fiber-Rich Foods: Foods high in dietary fiber, such as whole grains, fruits, and vegetables, can help regulate blood sugar levels and promote satiety. Include fiber-rich options in your meals.

5. Avoid Overeating: Be mindful of portion sizes to prevent overeating. Overconsumption can lead to weight gain and potentially hinder neurogenesis.

6. Snacking: If you need a snack between meals, opt for healthy choices like nuts, seeds, yogurt, or fresh fruit. Avoid sugary or processed snacks.

7. Hydration: Stay adequately hydrated throughout the day by drinking water. Dehydration can affect cognitive function and overall brain health.

8. Meal Timing for Exercise: If you engage in regular exercise, consider the timing of your meals in relation to your workouts. Eating a balanced meal or snack with carbohydrates and protein 1-2 hours before exercise can provide energy, while consuming a protein-rich meal or snack after exercise supports muscle recovery.

9. Time-Restricted Eating: Some research suggests that time-restricted eating, where you limit your daily eating to a specific window of time (e.g., 8 hours), may have benefits for brain health and metabolism. Consult with a healthcare professional before adopting this approach.

10. Evening Meals: Be cautious about heavy or high-calorie meals close to bedtime. Late-night eating can disrupt sleep, which is essential for brain health.

11. Mindful Eating: Practice mindful eating by savoring each bite, paying attention to hunger and fullness cues, and minimizing distractions during meals. Mindful eating can help you make healthier food choices and prevent overeating.

12. Individual Needs: Recognize that meal planning and timing can vary from person to person. Factors such as age, activity level, and personal preferences should inform your meal planning decisions.

CHAPTER 5

Neurogenesis Diet Recipes

5.1 Breakfast Options

Starting your day with a neurogenesis-friendly breakfast sets a positive tone for the rest of the day. Here are three delicious breakfast recipes that incorporate neurogenesis-promoting ingredients:

1. Blueberry and Almond Butter Oatmeal

Ingredients:

- 1/2 cup old-fashioned oats

- 1 cup almond milk (or your preferred milk)

- 1/2 cup fresh or frozen blueberries

- 1 tablespoon almond butter

- 1 tablespoon honey or maple syrup (optional)

- A pinch of cinnamon

- Chopped almonds for garnish

Instructions:

1. In a saucepan, combine oats and almond milk. Cook over medium heat, stirring occasionally, until the oats are tender and the mixture thickens (usually about 5-7 minutes).

2. Stir in the blueberries and almond butter. Cook for an additional 2-3 minutes until the blueberries are heated through.

3. If desired, sweeten with honey or maple syrup and sprinkle with a pinch of cinnamon.

4. Serve hot, garnished with chopped almonds for added crunch and nutrition.

2. Spinach and Mushroom Breakfast Scramble

Ingredients:

- 2 large eggs
- 1 cup fresh spinach, chopped
- 1/2 cup sliced mushrooms
- 1/4 cup diced onions
- 1 clove garlic, minced
- Olive oil for cooking
- Salt and pepper to taste

- Grated Parmesan cheese (optional)

Instructions:

1. In a skillet, heat a small amount of olive oil over medium heat. Add the diced onions and sauté until translucent.

2. Add the minced garlic and sliced mushrooms to the skillet. Cook until the mushrooms become tender and browned.

3. Add the chopped spinach to the skillet and cook until it wilts.

4. In a bowl, whisk the eggs and season with salt and pepper.

5. Pour the beaten eggs over the vegetables in the skillet. Gently scramble the eggs and mix them with the vegetables until fully cooked.

6. If desired, top with a sprinkle of grated Parmesan cheese before serving.

3. Avocado and Smoked Salmon Toast

Ingredients:

- 1 slice of whole-grain or sprouted grain bread

- 1/2 ripe avocado

- 2-3 slices of smoked salmon

- Sliced cucumber and cherry tomatoes for garnish

- Lemon juice for drizzling

- Fresh dill for garnish (optional)

- Salt and pepper to taste

Instructions:

1. Toast the slice of bread to your desired level of crispness.

2. While the bread is toasting, mash the ripe avocado in a bowl. Season it with a dash of lemon juice, salt, and pepper.

3. Once the toast is ready, spread the mashed avocado evenly on top.

4. Arrange the smoked salmon slices on the avocado.

5. Garnish with sliced cucumber, cherry tomatoes, and fresh dill.

6. Drizzle with a bit more lemon juice for added flavor.

These breakfast options not only taste great but also provide essential nutrients to support brain health and neurogenesis. Customize them to your preferences and enjoy a nutritious start to your day.

5.2 Lunch Ideas

For a neurogenesis-friendly lunch, focus on incorporating nutrient-dense ingredients and foods that support brain health. Here are three delicious lunch ideas that align with the principles of a Neurogenesis Diet:

1. Quinoa and Chickpea Salad

Ingredients:

- 1 cup cooked quinoa

- 1 cup cooked chickpeas (canned or pre-cooked)

- 1 cup chopped fresh spinach or kale

- 1/2 cup diced cucumber

- 1/2 cup cherry tomatoes, halved

- 1/4 cup chopped red onion

- 1/4 cup crumbled feta cheese (optional)

- 2 tablespoons extra-virgin olive oil

- 1 tablespoon lemon juice

- 1 clove garlic, minced

- Salt and pepper to taste

Instructions:

1. In a large bowl, combine cooked quinoa, chickpeas, chopped spinach or kale, cucumber, cherry tomatoes, and red onion.

2. In a small bowl, whisk together the extra-virgin olive oil, lemon

juice, minced garlic, salt, and pepper to create the dressing.

3. Pour the dressing over the salad and toss to coat all the ingredients evenly.

4. If desired, sprinkle crumbled feta cheese on top for added flavor.

5. Serve immediately or refrigerate for later use. This salad can be enjoyed warm or cold.

2. Salmon and Avocado Wrap

Ingredients:

- 1 whole-grain or spinach tortilla wrap

- 4 ounces cooked salmon (grilled or baked)

- 1/2 ripe avocado, sliced

- 1/4 cup mixed greens (e.g., arugula, baby spinach)

- Sliced red bell pepper

- Sliced red onion

- Greek yogurt or tzatziki sauce for drizzling

- Lemon wedges for squeezing

- Salt and pepper to taste

Instructions:

1. Lay the tortilla wrap flat on a clean surface.

2. Place the cooked salmon, sliced avocado, mixed greens, red bell pepper, and red onion in the center of the tortilla.

3. Drizzle Greek yogurt or tzatziki sauce over the ingredients.

4. Squeeze fresh lemon juice over the filling and season with salt and pepper.

5. Fold the sides of the tortilla inward, then roll it up tightly from the bottom to create a wrap.

6. Cut the wrap in half diagonally, if desired, and serve.

3. Lentil and Vegetable Soup

Ingredients:

- 1 cup dried green or brown lentils

- 4 cups vegetable broth

- 1 cup diced carrots

- 1 cup diced celery

- 1 cup diced onion

- 1 cup diced bell peppers (assorted colors)

- 2 cloves garlic, minced

- 1 teaspoon olive oil

- 1 teaspoon ground cumin

- 1/2 teaspoon turmeric

- Salt and pepper to taste

- Fresh parsley or cilantro for garnish (optional)

Instructions:

1. In a large pot, heat the olive oil over medium heat. Add the diced onion, garlic, and a pinch of salt. Sauté until the onions become translucent.

2. Stir in the diced carrots, celery, and bell peppers. Cook for a

few minutes until the vegetables begin to soften.

3. Add the lentils, vegetable broth, ground cumin, turmeric, salt, and pepper. Bring to a boil.

4. Reduce the heat to a simmer and cover the pot. Allow the soup to simmer for about 20-25 minutes, or until the lentils and vegetables are tender.

5. Taste and adjust seasoning as needed. If desired, garnish with fresh parsley or cilantro before serving.

These lunch ideas are not only delicious but also provide a balance of nutrients to support brain health and neurogenesis. Feel free to adapt them to your preferences and dietary requirements for a satisfying and nourishing midday meal.

5.3 Dinner Recipes

Dinner is an excellent opportunity to incorporate neurogenesis-promoting foods into your diet. Here are two flavorful dinner recipes that align with the principles of a Neurogenesis Diet:

1. Baked Salmon with Quinoa and Steamed Broccoli

Ingredients:

- 2 salmon fillets (6-8 ounces each)
- 1 cup quinoa, rinsed
- 2 cups water or vegetable broth
- 2 cups broccoli florets
- 1 lemon, thinly sliced
- 2 cloves garlic, minced
- 2 tablespoons olive oil

- 1 teaspoon dried thyme

- Salt and pepper to taste

- Fresh parsley for garnish (optional)

Instructions:

1. Preheat your oven to 375°F (190°C).

2. Place the salmon fillets on a baking sheet lined with parchment paper. Drizzle them with olive oil, and season with minced garlic, dried thyme, salt, and pepper.

3. Lay lemon slices over the salmon fillets.

4. Bake the salmon in the preheated oven for 15-20 minutes or until it flakes easily with a fork.

5. While the salmon is baking, rinse the quinoa under cold water. In a saucepan, bring 2 cups of water or vegetable broth to a boil. Add the quinoa, reduce heat to low, cover, and simmer for about 15 minutes, or until the liquid is absorbed and the quinoa is tender.

6. Steam the broccoli until it's bright green and tender, which usually takes about 5 minutes.

7. Serve the baked salmon over cooked quinoa, with steamed broccoli on the side. Garnish with fresh parsley, if desired.

2. Veggie Stir-Fry with Tofu and Brown Rice

Ingredients:

- 1 cup brown rice, cooked

- 8 ounces extra-firm tofu, cubed

- 2 cups mixed vegetables (e.g., bell peppers, broccoli, snap peas, carrots)

- 2 tablespoons low-sodium soy sauce or tamari

- 1 tablespoon rice vinegar

- 1 teaspoon sesame oil

- 1 clove garlic, minced

- 1/2 teaspoon fresh ginger, grated

- 1 tablespoon olive oil or vegetable oil

- Sesame seeds and chopped green onions for garnish (optional)

Instructions:

1. In a small bowl, whisk together soy sauce or tamari, rice vinegar, sesame oil, minced garlic, and grated ginger to make the stir-fry sauce.

2. In a large skillet or wok, heat the olive oil over medium-high heat. Add the cubed tofu and stir-fry until it becomes golden and crispy on all sides.

3. Remove the tofu from the skillet and set it aside.

4. In the same skillet, add a bit more oil if needed and stir-fry the mixed vegetables until they are tender-crisp, about 5-7 minutes.

5. Return the tofu to the skillet and pour the stir-fry sauce over the tofu and vegetables. Stir well to coat everything evenly

and heat for an additional 2-3 minutes.

6. Serve the tofu and vegetable stir-fry over cooked brown rice.

7. Garnish with sesame seeds and chopped green onions if desired.

5.4 Snacks and Smoothies

Here are a couple of neurogenesis-friendly snack and smoothie ideas:

1. Nut and Berry Trail Mix

Ingredients:

- 1/4 cup almonds

- 1/4 cup walnuts

- 1/4 cup dried blueberries or cranberries

- 1/4 cup dark chocolate chips (70% cocoa or higher)

- 1/4 cup pumpkin seeds

- 1/4 cup sunflower seeds

Instructions:

1. Mix all the ingredients together in a bowl.

2. Portion into small snack bags for easy, on-the-go snacking.

2. Blueberry and Spinach Smoothie

Ingredients:

- 1 cup fresh spinach leaves

- 1/2 cup frozen blueberries

- 1/2 banana

- 1/2 cup Greek yogurt or dairy-free yogurt

- 1 tablespoon almond butter

- 1 teaspoon honey or maple syrup (optional)

- 1 cup unsweetened almond milk or your preferred milk

Instructions:

1. Place all the ingredients in a blender.

2. Blend until smooth and creamy. If it's too thick, add more almond milk.

3. Taste and add honey or maple syrup if you prefer a sweeter smoothie.

4. Pour into a glass and enjoy as a snack or light meal.

These dinner recipes, snacks, and smoothies are not only delicious but also provide the nutrients needed to support brain health and neurogenesis. Feel free to customize them to suit your taste preferences and dietary requirements.

CHAPTER 6

Incorporating Lifestyle Changes

6.1 Exercise and Neurogenesis

Exercise is a powerful lifestyle factor that significantly influences neurogenesis and overall brain health. Engaging in regular physical activity can enhance cognitive function, stimulate the growth of new neurons, and support a healthier brain. Here's how exercise contributes to neurogenesis and some tips on incorporating it into your daily routine:

How Exercise Promotes Neurogenesis:

1. **Increased Blood Flow:** Exercise enhances blood flow to the brain, ensuring that brain cells receive an adequate supply of oxygen and nutrients necessary for neurogenesis.

2. **Release of Neurotrophic Factors:** Physical activity stimulates the release of neurotrophic factors like brain-derived neurotrophic factor (BDNF). BDNF plays a crucial role in the growth, survival, and maintenance of neurons.

3. **Reduced Inflammation:** Exercise has anti-inflammatory effects, which can protect existing brain cells from damage and promote a

conducive environment for neurogenesis.

4. **Stress Reduction:** Regular exercise helps manage stress and reduces the levels of stress hormones like cortisol. High levels of cortisol can inhibit neurogenesis, so stress reduction is beneficial.

5. **Enhanced Synaptic Plasticity:** Exercise can improve synaptic plasticity, the brain's ability to adapt and form new connections, which is closely linked to neurogenesis.

Tips for Incorporating Exercise into Your Routine:

1. **Choose Activities You Enjoy:** Find physical activities you genuinely enjoy, whether it's dancing, hiking, swimming, or

playing a sport. This makes it more likely that you'll stick with it.

2. **Start Slowly:** If you're new to exercise or haven't been active for a while, start with manageable activities and gradually increase intensity and duration. Consistency is key.

3. **Set Realistic Goals:** Establish achievable fitness goals to stay motivated. These could include walking a certain number of steps per day, increasing your weekly workout time, or learning a new exercise skill.

4. **Incorporate Variety:** Incorporate a variety of exercises into your routine to engage different muscle groups and keep things interesting.

This can also help prevent overuse injuries.

5. **Make It Social:** Exercise with friends or join group classes to make physical activity a social experience. The social aspect can add motivation and enjoyment.

6. **Create a Routine:** Set a regular exercise schedule that fits your lifestyle. Consistency in timing can help establish a habit.

7. **Combine Aerobic and Strength Training:** Incorporate both aerobic exercises (like jogging or cycling) and strength training (using weights or resistance bands) into your routine for comprehensive benefits.

8. **Practice Mindfulness:**
   Mindful movement practices like yoga and tai chi not only provide physical benefits but also support mental well-being and relaxation, which can enhance neurogenesis.

9. **Stay Hydrated:** Proper hydration is essential for overall health, including optimal brain function during exercise.

10. **Consult a Professional:** If you have underlying health conditions or concerns, consult with a healthcare provider or fitness expert before starting a new exercise regimen.

6.2 Sleep and Stress Management

Incorporating proper sleep and effective stress management strategies into your lifestyle is crucial for supporting neurogenesis and overall brain health. Both sleep and stress have profound effects on cognitive function and can either promote or hinder the growth of new neurons. Here's how to optimize these aspects of your life:

1. Sleep and Neurogenesis:

- **Sleep Quality:** Aim for 7-9 hours of quality sleep per night. Quality sleep includes sufficient time in deep and REM (rapid eye movement) sleep stages, which are critical for cognitive function and memory consolidation.

- **Consistent Sleep Schedule:** Try to go to bed and wake up at the same time every day, even on weekends. This helps regulate your body's internal clock.

- **Sleep Environment:** Create a comfortable sleep environment by keeping your bedroom cool, dark, and quiet. Invest in a comfortable mattress and pillows.

- **Limit Screen Time:** Reduce exposure to screens (phones, tablets, computers, TVs) before bedtime. The blue light emitted from screens can disrupt your circadian rhythm.

- **Avoid Heavy Meals and Stimulants:** Avoid heavy meals, caffeine, and alcohol close to bedtime, as they can interfere with sleep quality.

- **Relaxation Techniques:** Practice relaxation techniques such as deep breathing, progressive muscle relaxation, or meditation before bedtime to calm your mind and prepare for sleep.

- **Limit Naps:** While short naps can be rejuvenating, excessive daytime napping can disrupt nighttime sleep patterns. Keep naps to 20-30 minutes if needed.

2. Stress Management and Neurogenesis:

- **Identify Stressors:** Identify sources of stress in your life, whether they are related to work, relationships, or personal issues.

- **Mindfulness and Meditation:** Mindfulness practices and meditation can help reduce stress by promoting relaxation and increasing resilience to stressors.

- **Exercise:** Regular physical activity can be an effective stress reducer. Exercise releases endorphins, which are natural mood lifters.

- **Healthy Diet:** A well-balanced diet, including neurogenesis-promoting foods, can help regulate stress hormones and support overall mental well-being.

- **Time Management:** Organize your time and prioritize tasks to

reduce feelings of overwhelm.
Break larger tasks into smaller,
more manageable steps.

- **Seek Support:** Talk to friends,
  family, or a mental health
  professional if you're dealing
  with chronic stress or anxiety.
  Sometimes, sharing your
  feelings and experiences can be
  a tremendous relief.

- **Hobbies and Relaxation:**
  Engage in hobbies or activities
  that you enjoy and that help
  you relax. Whether it's reading,
  painting, or spending time in
  nature, these activities can be
  soothing.

- **Limit Exposure to Stressors:**
  If possible, limit exposure to
  ongoing stressors. This may
  involve setting boundaries,

reassessing commitments, or making necessary lifestyle changes.

- **Biofeedback and Relaxation Techniques:** Consider exploring biofeedback and relaxation techniques to gain better control over your body's response to stress.

- **Sleep and Stress:** Address sleep problems, as insufficient sleep can increase stress levels. Follow the sleep tips mentioned earlier to ensure adequate rest.

Stress and sleep are interconnected. Chronic stress can disrupt sleep, and poor sleep can exacerbate stress. By addressing both sleep and stress management, you create a positive feedback loop that supports neurogenesis and enhances overall cognitive function. Implementing these strategies may take time, but the benefits for your brain health and well-being are well worth the effort.

6.3 Cognitive Stimulation

Cognitive stimulation is a key component of maintaining and enhancing brain health, including supporting neurogenesis. Engaging in activities that challenge your brain, foster learning, and stimulate cognitive function can contribute to the growth of new neurons and the development of neural connections. Here are some strategies to incorporate cognitive stimulation into your daily life:

1. Lifelong Learning:

- **Read Regularly:** Make reading a habit. Explore a variety of genres, from fiction and non-fiction to magazines and academic papers. Reading exposes your brain to new ideas and vocabulary.

- **Learn a New Skill:** Challenge yourself by acquiring a new skill or hobby. This could be learning to play a musical instrument, speaking a new language, or taking up a craft.

- **Online Courses:** Take advantage of online courses and tutorials. Platforms like Coursera, edX, and Khan Academy offer a wide range of free or low-cost courses on diverse subjects.

- **Attend Workshops and Seminars:** Participate in workshops, seminars, or lectures in your area of interest. Local community centers, libraries, and universities often host such events.

2. Puzzles and Brain Games:

- **Crossword Puzzles:** Solve crossword puzzles to challenge your vocabulary and problem-solving skills. There are many crossword apps and books available.

- **Sudoku:** Sudoku puzzles engage logical thinking and number skills. They come in various difficulty levels, making them suitable for all levels of expertise.

- **Brain-Training Apps:** Explore brain-training apps like Lumosity, Elevate, or Peak, which offer a variety of games designed to enhance memory, attention, and cognitive flexibility.

3. Social Interaction:

- **Engage in Discussions:** Engage in conversations and discussions on a wide range of topics. Debate and share ideas with friends and family to stimulate critical thinking.

- **Join Clubs or Groups:** Join clubs or social groups that align with your interests. Book clubs, debate clubs, and hobbyist groups provide opportunities for meaningful social interaction and cognitive stimulation.

4. Creative Expression:

- **Write:** Keep a journal, write poetry, or work on a novel. Writing exercises your creativity, language skills, and self-expression.

- **Artistic Pursuits:** Engage in artistic activities like drawing, painting, or sculpting. These activities encourage creativity and spatial thinking.

- **Music:** Learning to play a musical instrument or composing music can stimulate both creativity and cognitive function.

5. Mindfulness Practices:

- **Meditation:** Regular meditation practice can improve focus, attention, and emotional regulation. It also supports overall brain health.

- **Yoga:** Yoga combines physical postures with mindfulness, promoting relaxation and mental clarity.

6. Travel and Exploration:

- **Travel:** Exploring new places, cultures, and cuisines can be a stimulating and enriching experience for the brain. Travel exposes you to new ideas and perspectives.

7. Stay Curious:

- **Ask Questions:** Cultivate curiosity by asking questions about the world around you. Be inquisitive and seek answers through research and exploration.

- **Problem-Solving:** Tackle real-life problems or challenges. This could involve anything from fixing household issues to volunteering for community initiatives.

Incorporating cognitive stimulation into your daily life not only supports neurogenesis but also contributes to a fulfilling and enriched existence. Remember that the brain benefits from novelty and variety, so try to diversify your cognitive activities to continually challenge your mental faculties.

CHAPTER 7

Monitoring Your Progress

Monitoring your progress while following a Neurogenesis Diet and implementing lifestyle changes is essential for gauging the effectiveness of your efforts and making necessary adjustments. Here are steps to help you track your diet, assess cognitive changes, and adapt your plan as needed:

7.1 Tracking Your Diet

1. **Food Journal:** Keep a detailed food journal to record what you eat and drink daily. Include

portion sizes, preparation
methods, and any neurogenesis-
promoting foods you consume.

2. **Meal Planning:** Plan your
   meals and snacks in advance.
   This allows you to ensure
   you're incorporating a variety
   of neurogenesis-promoting
   foods into your diet and
   maintaining a balanced
   approach.

3. **Nutrient Tracking Apps:**
   Consider using nutrient
   tracking apps or websites that
   can help you monitor your
   daily intake of essential
   nutrients. These tools can
   provide insights into your diet's
   nutritional profile.

4. **Regular Weigh-Ins:** If weight
   management is one of your

goals, weigh yourself regularly and track your progress. Remember that weight changes may take time to become apparent.

5. **Listen to Your Body:** Pay attention to how your body responds to different foods and dietary choices. Note any changes in energy levels, mood, digestion, and overall well-being.

7.2 Assessing Cognitive Changes

1. **Cognitive Testing:** Consider taking cognitive tests or assessments before and periodically during your neurogenesis-focused journey.

These assessments can help measure changes in cognitive function.

2. **Self-Reflection:** Self-assess your cognitive function regularly. Are you experiencing improvements in memory, concentration, problem-solving, or mental clarity? Note any changes in your mental abilities.

3. **Mood and Well-Being:** Monitor your mood and emotional well-being. Improved brain health often correlates with enhanced mood and reduced stress and anxiety.

4. **Sleep Quality:** Track your sleep patterns and quality. Adequate, restful sleep is crucial for cognitive function,

and improvements in sleep may indicate positive changes in your brain health.

7.3 Adjusting Your Plan

1. **Review Your Food Journal:** Periodically review your food journal to identify patterns and trends in your dietary habits. Are you consistently including neurogenesis-promoting foods?

2. **Consult a Healthcare Professional:** If you're not experiencing the desired cognitive improvements or if you encounter challenges with your diet or lifestyle changes, consult a healthcare provider or nutritionist for guidance.

3. **Modify Your Diet:** Based on your food journal and any advice from professionals, make adjustments to your diet. Consider adding new neurogenesis-promoting foods or altering your meal planning strategy.

4. **Evaluate Exercise Routine:** Assess your exercise routine. Are you being consistent with physical activity, and are you progressively challenging yourself? Adjust your exercise regimen as needed to ensure it aligns with your goals.

5. **Manage Stress and Sleep:** If stress or sleep issues persist, explore additional stress management techniques, mindfulness practices, or

adjustments to your sleep
routine.

6. **Set New Goals:** Continually set
new cognitive and lifestyle
goals. As you achieve
milestones, set higher targets to
continue improving brain
health and neurogenesis.

7. **Seek Support:** If you
encounter challenges or
setbacks, don't hesitate to seek
support from a healthcare
provider, nutritionist, or mental
health professional. They can
provide guidance and tailored
recommendations.

Progress can be gradual, and
individual results may vary. Be
patient with yourself, and celebrate
small victories along the way. Regular
monitoring and adaptability are key to

successfully maintaining a Neurogenesis Diet and supporting your long-term brain health and cognitive function.

Made in United States
Troutdale, OR
05/06/2024

19692103R10056